HPV

A GUIDEBOOK TO INFECTION WITH HUMAN PAPILLOMAVIRUS AND HOW TO

Fight Back!

Laura F. McKain, MD

Why I Wrote This Book

In short, there's nothing out there quite like this book and it simply <u>needed</u> to be written. The long version is, well, a bit longer. Over my years of clinical practice, I spent hours and hours in the colposcopy room at my doctor's office, caring for women infected with human papillomavirus (HPV). I evaluated and treated women with abnormal Pap tests, used cryotherapy to remove genital warts, and performed LEEP biopsies to remove precancerous cells from the cervix - all symptoms of HPV. The fact is, if you found yourself in my colposcopy room, it was probably due to HPV. Sadly, this room saw a lot of use. There were often scheduling conflicts for this room because so many women needed care.

Naturally, much of the conversation in the colposcopy room was HPV-oriented. Many women were surprised to know that their abnormal Pap results were related to HPV and struggled to understand the meaning of their results. They wondered how they got the virus, from whom they'd gotten it, and how long they had been infected. There never seemed to be enough time to answer all of the women's questions. There certainly was not enough time to provide in-depth instruction in the biology of HPV and (more importantly) how the body fights it. In my sessions with patients, I generally focused on the risks and benefits of medical treatment, what basic health measures to take, and the importance of follow-up visits. This approach was not very holistic and did not encompass everything that is known about the natural history of HPV. There simply was not enough time.

So, I wrote this book to give women a better understanding of this infection, and what they need to know to cope successfully with and beat HPV! I want women to <u>know their enemy</u>— to have the knowledge they need about the biology of HPV and the factors that contribute to healing. The fact is, getting well and staying well after an HPV infection is not just about getting the right medical care.

Please, don't misunderstand me! Getting medical care <u>is</u> <u>critical</u> in detecting and treating precancerous changes caused by HPV—you should never skip that step! But, there are so many other things women can and should do to increase their chances of a positive outcome.

I never had enough time to tell women everything they needed to know about HPV. Your health care provider probably doesn't either. **That is the purpose of this book.** I have taken the time here to say it all.

I am going to teach you a lot about HPV infection through the course of this book. First, you will find out what HPV is, the problems it causes, and how it is diagnosed. You'll learn about the applicable medical treatments and care options, as well as the biology of how your body naturally fights HPV.

The second part of this book is all about helping your body fight HPV. I will teach you about behaviors, nutritional factors, and self-care that can dramatically increase your chances of clearing away your HPV. The goal here is to empower you, so you don't feel like a victim of this virus. I have even included a few real-life stories of women and their battles with HPV. Hopefully, these stories will help you to see that there really **are** things you can do to get better.

I suggest you read this book from cover to cover. In the first part of the book, I want you to find out as much about HPV as possible. Identify the information that matches your personal situation. Learn the natural history of HPV and the medical treatments that can treat the conditions caused by HPV.

In the second part of the book, ask yourself lots of questions. What haven't you been doing that you should? What are you doing that you shouldn't? What can you do better? I have provided a wealth of advice to you in this section. Read it with the purpose of identifying specific actions you can take to ensure the best possible outcome. Don't just accept an HPV infection…

FIGHT BACK!

Table of Contents

PART ONE:

All about HPV Infection

Chapter 1: What Is HPV?

The human papillomavirus (HPV) is the most common sexually transmitted infection. There are more than 150 types of HPV. More than 40 of them can be easily transmitted through direct skin-to-skin contact during vaginal, anal, or oral sex. Most of the time, when someone becomes infected with HPV, it goes away on its own and causes no problems at all. However, sometimes the HPV infection persists and can cause significant health problems like genital warts and cancer.

The "genotypes", (or just the "types") of HPV that infect the genitals can be categorized as either low-risk or high-risk. There are roughly 12 types that are known as low-risk because they do not have the potential to cause cancer. These types can, however, cause genital warts or minor cell changes on the cervix. Types 6 and 11 are responsible for nearly 90% of genital warts.

There are more than a dozen high-risk types of HPV that have the potential to cause persistent infections. Over time, these can lead to cancer of the cervix, vulva, vagina, anus, and penis. Virtually all cervical cancers are caused by high-risk type HPV infections. Types 16 and 18 are responsible for 70% of all cervical cancers.

HPV Genotypes

LOW RISK	HIGH RISK
6, 11, 40, 42, 43, 44, 53, 54, 61, 72, 73, 81	16, 18, 31, 33, 35, 39, 45, 51, 52, 56, 59, 66, 68
• Genital warts • Low-grade cervical abnormalities	• Low-grade cervical abnormalities • High-grade cervical abnormalities • Cervical cancer • Other genital cancers

How common is HPV infection?

The short answer is VERY. At any given time, 43% of women aged 14-59 show symptoms of HPV infections. Over the course of their lifetime, 80% of all women get HPV. It is important to keep in mind that although HPV is common, cervical cancer is rare. The American Cancer Society predicts that roughly 13,000 women will be diagnosed with cervical cancer in the U.S. this year, and about 4,000 of them will die from it. That equates to 7.7 new cases of cervical cancer per 100,000 women.

Nonetheless, detecting and treating HPV disease is what keeps the incidence of cervical cancer in check. Thus, it is important for all women to be aware of

HPV and to take appropriate steps to prevent serious consequences.

What are the risk factors for HPV?

There are a number of risk factors associated with the development of an HPV infection, especially for persistent HPV and the development of cervical cancer. These include:

- Having many sexual partners
- Having a partner who has had many sexual partners
- Starting to have sex at a young age
- Current or previous use of cigarettes
- Oral contraceptive use
- Immunosuppression
- Co-infection with other sexually transmitted diseases

What kind of health problems does HPV cause?

Most people who become infected with HPV show absolutely no symptoms and their immune system eventually just clears the infection without any consequences. But there are certain types of HPV that can cause disease soon after infection and some types that can persist for years and cause very serious problems.

Genital Warts

As mentioned earlier, low-risk HPV types 6 and 11 are responsible for most cases of genital warts. Genital warts appear as bumps that can be raised or flat and have surfaces that are either smooth or ragged like a cauliflower. There may be one wart or many, and they can be tiny or astonishingly large. Usually, your health care provider can make a diagnosis just by looking at your warts.

Here are some additional facts:

- At any given time, about 1% of sexually active people show evidence of genital warts.

- Two-thirds of people who have sexual contact with someone with genital warts will develop warts themselves.

- The exact incubation time of genital warts is not known, but it has been estimated to be anywhere from 3 weeks to 8 months (or even longer).

- As many as 20% of people with genital warts have some other sexually transmitted infection, so it is important to get medical care if you think you have genital warts.

The types of HPV that cause warts are considered to be "benign" strains, meaning they do not ever cause cancer. Genital warts often go away all by themselves, usually within the first 2 years of appearing. There <u>are</u> treatments for genital warts (see Chapter 3) that can make the warts disappear. Unfortunately, these options are often only temporarily effective.

Women who have HPV during pregnancy may worry that this will harm their unborn child. In most cases, HPV doesn't affect a developing fetus. An HPV infection, manifested as genital warts, does not usually change the way a woman is cared for during pregnancy.

Sometimes, during pregnancy, a combination of surging hormones and the suppression of the immune system can allow genital warts to grow in size and number. The risk of transmitting HPV to your baby is so small (just 0.05%), so vaginal delivery is nearly always recommended (even if the mother has a large number of warts). In rare circumstances, genital warts can grow to such a size that they obstruct the birth canal, making a cesarean section necessary. More often, if the size of warty growths becomes a problem, your health care provider will undertake aggressive treatment to remove them before your baby is born.

Cervical Disease

High-risk type HPV infections can cause pre-cancerous conditions or full-blown cancer of the cervix. It usually takes years (or even decades) for a high-risk HPV infection to turn into cervical cancer. In one study by the National Cancer Institute, it was found that about 10% of women with HPV types 16 or 18 developed advanced, high-grade cervical disease within three years; 20% did so in 10 years. Pap tests are aimed at identifying precancerous changes so that they can be treated - long before they turn into cancer.

The surface of the cervix is covered by a layer of cells called the epidermis. The epidermis lies on top of a basement membrane that separates it from the dermis below. HPV infections occur when tiny breaks in the epidermis called "micro-abrasions" allow the virus to access the cells just above the basement membrane. Most of the time, the immune system fights off the HPV infection. However, when the infection persists, HPV can disrupt cell growth and result in abnormal cells known as cervical intraepithelial neoplasia (CIN). When just the lower third of the epidermis is involved, this is called CIN 1. About 80% of the time, CIN 1 will go away on its own.

CIN caused by persistent infection with high-risk types of HPV can progress to high-grade abnormalities and involve more of the epidermis. This can result in CIN 2 and CIN 3-type lesions. If CIN 3 is left untreated, it can break through the basement membrane and become invasive cervical cancer. Cervical cancer screening programs are aimed at preventing cervical cancer by identifying women with CIN 2 and CIN 3 lesions so they can be treated before these lesions progress to cancer.

Progression of Cervical Disease Following HPV Infection

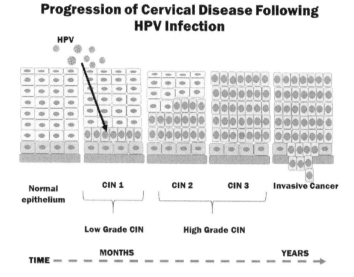

Other Cancers

HPV has been associated with a number of other cancers, as described below:

Vulvar Cancer

Research indicates that infection with high-risk HPV is a risk factor for vulvar cancer or malignancy of the outer portions of the female genitals. According to the American Cancer Society, there are about 4,850 new cases of vulvar cancer in the United States each year. Like cervical cancer, vulvar cancer forms slowly over many years and is usually preceded by precancerous changes. Symptoms of vulvar cancer may include:

- Itching that doesn't go away

- Pain and tenderness in one spot in the vulvar area

- Skin changes, such as color changes or thickening

- A lump, wart-like bumps, or an open sore (ulcer)

Vaginal Cancer

Cancer of the vagina is fairly rare—the incidence is 0.7 cases per 100,000 women. About 70% of vaginal cancers are squamous cell cancers related to HPV. Again, precancerous changes precede invasive vaginal cancer and can be identified during an exam (and sometimes even by a Pap test).

Oral Cancer

The same types of HPV that infect the genital areas can also infect the mouth and throat. This is called "oral HPV." High-risk types of HPV can cause cancers of the head and neck. Low-risk types of oral HPV can cause warts in the mouth or throat. In most cases, HPV infections of all types go away before they cause any health problems.

Chapter 2: How Do You Know if You Have HPV?

This chapter discusses the different ways HPV is diagnosed.

Genital Warts

People with genital warts usually notice the growths themselves. However, sometimes genital warts are found by a health care provider during an exam. Your health care provider can usually make a diagnosis by just looking at the warts.

If you are diagnosed with genital warts, your health care provider will probably ask you to get a blood test for syphilis because, in some rare cases, syphilis can also cause warty growths. It is important to rule out syphilis because, unlike genital warts, it can have serious health consequences if left untreated. It is rarely necessary to take biopsies of genital warts. Also, as I mentioned before, genital warts are not caused by the types of HPV that can cause cancer (so cultures are not helpful).

Having genital warts means you have been exposed to one sexually transmitted infection and possibly others. You could also be infected with a high-risk strain of HPV that could cause cervical disease, or even have another type of infection like chlamydia or gonorrhea. It is a good idea to talk to your health care provider about testing for other sexually transmitted infections, such as:

- Syphilis
- HIV
- Chlamydia
- Gonorrhea
- Cervical cancer screening (if appropriate)
- Hepatitis

Abnormal Pap Test

Many women find out that they have an HPV infection when a routine cervical cancer screening shows abnormal results. Remember, cervical cancer screening is aimed at detecting high-grade CIN (CIN 2 and 3) which, if untreated, could turn into cervical cancer.

What is a Pap Test?

The Pap test was introduced by Dr. George Papanicolaou in the 1950s as a screening test for cervical cancer. It is a very simple test in which a sample of cervical cells is examined under a microscope to detect abnormal cells—particularly cells that have been infected with HPV and undergone precancerous changes. A Pap sample is collected during a pelvic exam. Your health care provider places a speculum into your vagina so they can see your cervix and samples cells from the surface of the cervix by sweeping it with a brush or spatula. The cells are then either put onto a slide (the old-fashioned method) or swished into a liquid to be sent to a lab. Liquid-based Pap samples can be used not only to examine cervical cells, but to test for other conditions, such as HPV, chlamydia, and gonorrhea.

Note, however, just because these tests can be done from a Pap specimen does not mean that they have automatically been done. Always ask your health care provider what tests will be done on your cervical specimen.

The following table summarizes the most current recommendations by the American Congress of Obstetricians and Gynecologists for Pap tests. One thing to note is that Pap testing is not recommended until age 21, even if a young woman is sexually active. Although young women do become infected with HPV, serious cervical disease is very, very uncommon. Most HPV infections are transient, and doing Pap tests in women younger than 21 would lead to many needless evaluations and procedures. However, although women younger than 21 do not need Pap tests, they do need gynecological care, testing for other sexually transmitted diseases, and contraception!

Cervical Cancer Screening Guidelines

Age	American Congress of Ob/Gyn 2009
<21	No Screening
21-29	Pap every 2 years HPV test not recommended
30-65	Pap every 3 years if 3 consecutive normal results Co-testing appropriate
> 65	After 3 normal screening results and no abnormal results in the previous 10 years, screening may be discontinued
After a hysterectomy	May discontinue if the hysterectomy was for a benign reason

What do the results of a Pap test mean?

Negative for Intraepithelial Lesion or Malignancy (NILM)

This result means that your Pap test was normal. The cytologist did not find any abnormal-looking cells, and particularly nothing to suggest the presence of CIN. It is important to note, however, that it is entirely possible to be infected with HPV and have a normal Pap test. For this reason, it is now recommended that women 30 and older get both a Pap test and a test for HPV. I will explain more about this later in the book.

12

Atypical Squamous Cells of Undetermined Significance (ASC-US)

This means that the cytologist who read your Pap test saw some cells that were funny-looking, but not obviously abnormal. If your Pap test is read this way, the next step is usually to undertake an HPV test to look for infection with high-risk HPV. If you are found to have high-risk HPV, your health care provider will probably want you to follow-up with a test called a colposcopy to evaluate whether you have high-grade CIN (CIN 2 or 3).

Women with an ASC-US Pap test AND a positive high-risk HPV infection have about a 5% chance of having high-grade CIN. It is essential to undertake the additional evaluations.

Low-Grade Squamous Intraepithelial Lesion (LSIL)

If your Pap test is read as LSIL, then it is likely that you have an HPV infection. This could just be an infection with low-risk HPV, but it could also be an infection with low-risk HPV that is causing CIN 1.

Alternatively, this could be a high-risk HPV infection (that may or may not be associated with CIN). There is about a 5% chance of having high-grade CIN when your Pap test is read as LSIL. Your health care provider will usually want you to follow-up with a colposcopy to look for high-grade CIN. Remember that most HPV infections, even those with high-risk

HPV, are temporary. If you have an LSIL Pap result and you are very young, your health care provider may want to wait a while before recommending a colposcopy.

You may wonder whether you should have a test for high-risk HPV if your Pap is read as LSIL. Probably not, because it is very, very likely that the test will be positive and knowing this result won't change your doctor's recommendations.

High-Grade squamous Intraepithelial Lesion (HSIL)

If your Pap test is read as HSIL, then it means the cytologist saw some abnormal cells that could be associated with high-grade CIN. Your health care provider will likely want you to follow up with a colposcopy.

This test result means you have a high risk of high-grade CIN. While this may seem scary, remember that this test result gives you an opportunity to get treatments that can prevent you from developing cervical cancer.

Other Findings

The most common findings on Pap tests have been discussed above. However, there are other ways your Pap may be reported. These include:

- Atypical Squamous Cells of Undetermined Significance (ASC-H) – Cannot exclude high-grade squamous intraepithelial lesion

- Atypical glandular cells (AGC)

- Squamous cell carcinoma

- Adenocarcinoma in situ (AIS)

- Adenocarcinoma

These are all rare, but they are serious findings that require additional cancer tests.

Positive HPV Test

HPV tests can detect infection with the high-risk strains of HPV which are capable of causing cancer. There is also a test that that specifically detects infection with HPV types 16 and 18. These two high-risk HPV types are responsible for about 70% of cervical cancers.

Testing for high-risk HPV is useful when a Pap test shows atypical cells (ASC-US results). If this Pap test is associated with a high-risk HPV infection, further evaluation for high-grade CIN is recommended.

Current guidelines suggest that women 30 years of age and older should be screened with "co-testing". This means that they should have both a Pap test and a high-risk HPV test. This combined screening is more sensitive than a Pap alone for finding women who may have a high grade CIN. Furthermore, women who have both a negative Pap test and a negative high-risk HPV test have an incredibly small chance of cervical cancer (or of developing cervical cancer in the following five years). This risk is so small that cervical cancer screening does not need to be repeated for 3-5 years if both tests are negative. Yay!

If co-testing is done, and your Pap test is normal (NILM), but your high-risk HPV test is positive, then you are at increased risk of future development of high-grade CIN; you should repeat these tests in a year. In at least 50% of women, their HPV infection will clear away during this year. If repeat testing shows that their HPV infection has not cleared, you should have a colposcopy to see whether or not you have developed high-grade CIN.

Another strategy for women with normal Pap results but a positive high-risk HPV test is to determine if the infection is caused by HPV types 16 or 18. Types 16 and 18 are the strains least likely to go away on their own and most commonly associated with cervical cancer. If either of these two strains are present, evaluation with a colposcopy should be done right away. If you have high-risk HPV but test negative for types 16 and 18, its more likely the infection will resolve on its own testing should be repeated in one year, as described above.

Because HPV infection is very common in women under 30, co-testing is not recommended.

In 2014, the FDA approved a stand-alone HPV screening test for women aged 25 and older. This test, the Roche Cobias test, detects whether any high-risk HPV is present and whether this HPV is either type 16 or 18. Professional organizations have not yet embraced this new test, so this method of screening has not yet been widely adopted.

Colposcopy

Colposcopy is the gold-standard test that determines if high-grade CIN or cervical cancer is present. During the procedure, a speculum is placed into the vagina so your cervix can be seen. A device called a

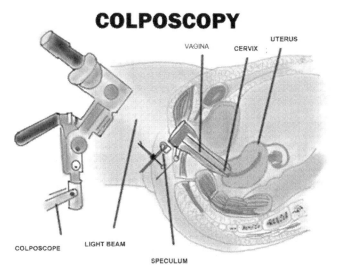

COLPOSCOPY

colposcope is used to shine a light onto the cervix so that it can be inspected through the magnifying scope. During colposcopy your health care provider may paint your cervix with a dilute solution of vinegar, which makes abnormal cells easier to see. Abnormal areas will be sampled with a small instrument that snips off a tiny piece of tissue. This tissue, known as a biopsy, will be sent off for inspection under a microscope by a pathologist. The pathologist will determine if CIN or cervical cancer is present. It usually takes from a few days to a week to get your pathology report. Once it is available, your health care provider will review this pathology report with you.

Chapter 3: How is HPV Disease Treated?

When an HPV infection causes disease, active treatment is often recommended, particularly if high-grade CIN has been found. Treatment is also available for lesser diseases like genital warts. The treatments recommended by your health care provider are an important way of fighting back against HPV!

Treating Genital Warts

Remember that warts are not worrisome, medically speaking. They do not lead to cancer. The reasons for treating warts are cosmetic, and to reduce symptoms. Remember, while treatments can get rid of your warts, this may only be temporary. People often have recurrences of genital warts.

Even without treatment, however, genital warts often resolve on their own. In fact, about 80% of the time, warts go away by themselves within 24 months.

Available treatments fall into three categories: patient-applied medications, health care provider-applied medications, and surgical treatments. Note that all of these treatments involve a health care provider. Over-the-counter treatments for warts are not meant to be used in the genital area. (Never, ever!)

Patient-Applied Medicines

Prescription medications that you apply yourself are often preferred because they can be used at home and only require follow-up from a health care provider if they are not effective. In order for them to work best, you have to be able to identify the warts that need treatment, be able to reach them to apply medicine, and be willing to stick to your treatment regimen. It is important to know that using more of these medicines than recommended (or using them more often than recommended) is not going to make your warts go away faster. In fact, doing this increases your chance of severe side effects. In other words, only use these medications as directed!

Podofilox

Podofilox is a drug that destroys warts by disrupting cell division. It comes as either a liquid solution that you apply with a cotton swab or a gel that you apply with your fingers directly to the warts. It must be applied twice a day for three consecutive days, followed by 4 days without any therapy. These one-week cycles can be repeated up to four times. It is very common to experience mild or moderate pain during treatment, and the area may become inflamed.

Imiquimod

This is a topical treatment that works by stimulating the immune system to produce substances such as interferon and cytokines that work to promote clearance of genital warts. This medication is applied three times a week (such as Monday, Wednesday, and Friday) at bedtime. It should be left on the skin for at least 6-10 hours and then washed away with soap and water. It is very common for Imiquimod to cause an inflammatory reaction, so be sure to carefully follow the instructions about washing off the medicine and taking rest days! If you develop a severe inflammation with sores, blisters, or ulcerations of the skin, you may need to take a break from treatment. Imiquimod may be used for up to 16 weeks. However, if warts persist, you will need to meet with your doctor to discuss other options.

Sinecatechins

Sinecatechin ointment is the first botanical drug ever approved by the FDA. Extracted from green tea, sinecatechins contain antioxidants and related substances that can help heal your infection. This ointment is applied three times a day for up to 16 weeks. Minor side effects include burning and itching.

Heath Care Provider-Applied Medicines

You must receive these treatments at your health care provider's office. It may take multiple visits before your warts are all gone.

Podophyllin

Podophyllin resin is applied directly to each wart by your health care provider. It is important that the area be completely dry before you dress (If

Podophyllin contacts your healthy skin, it can cause a burn). You will be instructed to wash off the Podophyllin in 1-4 hours. Local irritation is common. Treatment is repeated weekly until your warts have cleared.

Trichloroacetic acid (TCA)

TCA has corrosive properties which destroy the proteins in the warty tissue. This destruction can extend beyond the superficial wart and kill the underlying infection. When the liquid is applied directly to the warts, they immediately take on a frosted appearance. Your health care provider may apply petroleum jelly to the surrounding tissue to protect it from the TCA. Treatment is often associated with temporary pain and burning. If your pain is severe, soap or baking soda can be used to neutralize the acid. An average of 8-10 weekly treatments are typically required to treat genital warts. This treatment is often used during pregnancy.

Surgical Treatments

Many surgical treatments are available to treat your genital warts. They provide quick results but do not always eradicate your infection. Recurrence of genital warts is not uncommon after surgical treatment.

Cryotherapy

Cryotherapy is a relatively inexpensive method of treatment, and has high success rates (around 70-80%) within the first 2-3 treatments. The application of nitrous oxide or liquid nitrogen causes permanent tissue damage to your warts. Blistering or ulceration may occur before the treated warts slough off. Because the treatment is lesion-focused, it does not affect subclinical infection in the surrounding areas. This is the treatment of choice during pregnancy.

Excision

Warts can be removed with a surgical scalpel or by electro surgery. This can be done in your health care provider's office or in a surgery center. Patients are given a local numbing medication. This approach may be used when warts are very large or have recurred after other treatments have been used. Risks include bleeding and infection.

Laser

Laser treatment is used for extensive or recurrent warts. A beam of light containing intense energy is used to vaporize the warty tissues. The laser can be used very precisely. This treatment is virtually bloodless because the laser cauterizes small blood vessels as the tissues are treated. Laser treatment is usually undertaken at a surgical center. You may be given general anesthesia to put you completely to sleep during the procedure. There can be significant pain after this treatment, especially if large areas are treated. Healing can take 2-4 weeks.

Treating Cervical Disease

As previously discussed, cervical diseases caused by HPV include:

- HPV infection without evidence of precancerous changes
- Low-grade CIN (CIN 1)
- High-grade CIN (CIN 2 and 3)
- Invasive cervical cancer

Cervical cancer screening is aimed at identifying precancerous lesions so they can be treated before they become invasive cervical cancers. The best treatment for your precancerous lesions will be determined by your health care provider, taking into account your medical history, the size of the lesion(s), the risk of progression to cancer, and other factors. Let's look at the different treatment options, according to the severity of the cervical disease.

Treating HPV infection and CIN 1

If a woman's tests show that she has an HPV infection, or if her infection has resulted in low-grade CIN or CIN 1, the chances are very good that both of these conditions will resolve without treatment. Only about 10 to 15% of CIN 1 lesions will progress to high-grade dysplasia over the next couple of years. Therefore, as long as a woman is responsible about following up with her doctor, the best thing to do is to wait to see what happens. If the woman follows up as directed, the chance of jumping from CIN 1 to invasive cancer in a short period of time is practically zero.

Your health care provider will probably ask you to come back in 12 months for another Pap test and, depending upon your age, possibly an HPV test. It is critical that you keep this follow-up appointment.

Will you be prescribed any medication while waiting? No, because there really isn't a medication to treat this condition.

Does this mean you don't have to do anything? No! In fact, Part Two of this book focuses on the many things you CAN do to increase your odds of clearing an HPV infection and helping your CIN 1 to regress.

Treating CIN 2 and CIN 3

Your risk of developing cervical cancer dramatically increases if you are diagnosed with CIN 2 or CIN 3, so some type of treatment is usually recommended. However, there is one exception:

Adolescents and young women with CIN 2 (Age 13-21)

The rate of regression of CIN 2 in young women is twice that of older women, so it is reasonable to observe women aged 13-21 with CIN 2 for up to 24 months, rather than proceeding directly to treatment. Colposcopy is then performed every 6 months. If the

CIN 2 lesion persists or progresses, treatment is recommended.

For women older than 21, treatment is recommended immediately.

LEEP

LEEP (loop electrosurgical excision procedure) is the most common treatment for CIN 2 and CIN 3. This procedure is done in your health care provider's office. A speculum is placed into your vagina, so your

LEEP
Loop Electrosurgical Excision Procedure

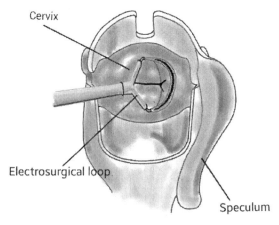

cervix is visible. Your doctor injects your cervix with a local numbing medicine and then uses a fine wire loop (with electricity flowing through it) to remove the abnormal cells from your cervix. This tissue will be sent to a pathologist to be inspected under a microscope to be sure that there is no evidence of invasive cancer.

It takes a while after a LEEP treatment for your cervix to heal. You must not put anything in the vagina—no tampons, no douching, no sex—for 4 weeks. You will have some bleeding and discharge during the healing process. You doctor will give you instructions about calling back if the bleeding is excessively heavy.

LEEP is about 98% effective at removing abnormal cells, but it may not completely cure your HPV infection. It is very, very important that you go back for follow-up visits according to your doctor's recommended schedule.

LEEP has been associated with pregnancy complications in some women. Most women do not have any problems, but some do experience increased risks of pregnancy loss and pre-term birth. It is important that you tell your obstetric care provider if you have had a LEEP treatment because they may want to monitor you more closely.

Conization

Conization, often called a cold knife cone, or cone biopsy, is the removal of a cone-shaped portion of the cervix with a scalpel. It can provide a deeper sample of the cervix, including better sampling of the canal of the cervix. This procedure is done in an operating room under general anesthesia.

Just like with a LEEP biopsy, the tissue removed will be examined under the microscope by the pathologist. You should put nothing in the vagina (no tampons, douching, or sex) for 4-6 weeks after the procedure. There is a risk of bleeding, and you will be given instructions on what to do if it is very heavy. Also, there is a risk of pregnancy complications, specifically of an incompetent cervix (which means that your cervix may not be strong enough to keep your baby in your womb). Your obstetric health care provider will want to monitor your pregnancy more closely after a conization.

Ablative procedures

It is worth mentioning two other procedures sometimes used in treating high-grade CIN, cryotherapy, and laser ablation. Both of these procedures destroy—or ablate—the abnormal cells on the surface of the cervix. Cryotherapy uses liquid nitrogen to freeze the cervix. This can be done in your health care provider's office in just a few minutes. Laser ablation is done in an operating room where a laser is used to vaporize the abnormal cells.

Most professional organizations favor excisional treatments (LEEP and conization) because they remove tissue in a way that allows for microscopic inspection for invasive cancer by a pathologist. Ablative procedures do not allow for further inspection of the removed tissue. It is important that you talk to your health care provider about the risks and benefits of all of these procedures so you can choose the treatment that is the best for you.

Hysterectomy

If a woman has CIN 3 or recurrent CIN 3 (and she does not want any more children), she may be offered a hysterectomy, which is the removal of the uterus and cervix. The doctor must be very certain that she does not have an invasive or micro-invasive cancer before doing a hysterectomy, so he or she may do a LEEP or conization first.

A hysterectomy is a major surgery and carries with it risks of complications such as bleeding, infection, and damage to internal organs like the bowel and bladder. It usually requires hospitalization and longer recovery times than the other procedures discussed. Also, removing the uterus and cervix does not completely negate the risk of cancer due to HPV. After a hysterectomy for CIN, women still need to get Pap tests for several years, at least.

Invasive Cervical Cancer

There are many different approaches to treating invasive cervical cancer; an entire book could written on this subject. I will try to provide a high-level overview of some of your options.

Your treatment will depend on a number of factors, such as:

- Your cancer stage—how deep and how far the cancer has invaded

- The cell type of your tumor

- Your age and other general health factors

If you are diagnosed with cervical cancer, you will likely be referred to a specialist called a gynecologic oncologist. Other doctors, such as those who specialize in radiation therapy, may also be involved in your care.

Very Early Stage (minimal invasion)

If your cancer is only micro-invasive or minimally invasive, it may be treated and cured with surgery alone. Approaches may include:

- Conization

- Simple hysterectomy—removal of the uterus and cervix

- Radical hysterectomy—removal of the cervix, uterus, tubes, and ovaries, as well as the accompanying lymph glands.

Early or Later Stages (deeper invasion or spread)

Your treatment will be more involved and may require a combination of several of the treatments below:

- Radiation therapy

- Simultaneous radiation therapy and chemotherapy
- A radical hysterectomy with or without radiation therapy
- Chemotherapy followed by surgery

Mikayla's Fight – Genital Warts

Mikayla first noticed her bumps in the shower. They just felt like tiny fleshy growths—there were about five or six of them. She tried to look at the area with a mirror, but it was really hard to see down there. She remembered learning about genital warts in a high school health class and had a sinking feeling about what might be happening to her. She decided it was time to visit the student health clinic.

The nurse practitioner confirmed her fears. She told Mikayla that their center had seen a number of genital wart cases on campus recently. She asked Mikayla whether or not she had been practicing safe sex (she had) and took some test samples with a cotton swab for gonorrhea and chlamydia. She also told Mikayla she wanted to do a blood test for syphilis and HIV, just as a precaution.

The nurse practitioner recommended that Mikayla try a medication, TCA, that would be applied right there in the office, that day. She asked Mikayla to check back with her in a week's time. Mikayla was relieved that there was something that could be done immediately to help her condition. She agreed to be treated.

The nurse practitioner applied the TCA. It burned like crazy at first, but after about 10 minutes Mikayla's

pain diminished to a minor stinging sensation.
Mikayla was instructed to wash the medicine off with
soap and water before bed and return in a week. She
went back to her dorm room feeling miserable, dirty,
and ashamed. She skipped all of her classes that day.

That evening, her boyfriend Trey stopped by. He
could tell right away that something was wrong. After
he pressed her about it, Mikayla told him the whole
story. Trey denied ever having had warts but
confessed that a previous girlfriend of his did.

Mikayla was furious! How could he not tell her this?
Trey was apologetic and said he hadn't thought it was
an issue. He had never had any problems himself and
had always used condoms, both with his old
girlfriend and with Mikayla.

Trey and Mikayla got on the internet together and
quickly realized that condoms do not provide perfect
protection. Trey promised to go to the student health
center the next day to get himself checked out.

The next week, Mikayla attended her follow-up
appointment. The nurse practitioner said all of
Mikayla's other STD tests were negative. She looked
at the warts and said they were considerably smaller.
She applied more TCA to Mikayla's warts. The
burning was less painful this time—certainly
tolerable.

Mikayla had a ton of questions. She had read that
HPV could cause cervical cancer and asked if she

should be getting a Pap test. The nurse practitioner said that because Mikayla was only 19, it was not recommended. First of all, the type of HPV that causes warts does not cause cervical cancer. Second of all, even if Mikayla did have other types of HPV, it was incredibly unlikely that she had any cervical disease at her young age because it takes years and years for HPV infection to progress to cancer. In young women like Mikayla, HPV infections usually go away on their own, so it was best for her to wait until she turned 21 to start getting Pap tests.

Mikayla told the nurse practitioner about Trey, and how his previous girlfriend had warts though Trey didn't. She said that Trey had come to the student health center for examination, but they hadn't found any warts on him.

Mikayla wanted to know if it was likely that she'd gotten her warts from Trey. The nurse practitioner said it was possible that Trey was a carrier and that Mikayla had gotten them from him. However, Mikayla could also have gotten her warts from a previous partner—there was no way to know for sure. She advised that Mikayla abstain from sex until her warts were gone and that she continue to practice safe sex using condoms. She also told Mikayla that this infection was now a part of her sexual history and that she should always be honest with future partners about it. Mikayla hated that thought but knew it was only fair.

The nurse practitioner also talked about the HPV vaccine, which Mikayla had never received. Her pediatrician had talked to her about it before leaving for college, but Mikayla had never bothered to go back for another appointment. She assumed that it was too late now, but the nurse practitioner explained that though the vaccine covers both strains of HPV that cause warts (too late for that!), it also protects against HPV strains that cause cervical cancer (maybe not too late!). The newest formulation, Gardasil 9, covers more cancer-causing strains than ever, and it might not be too late for Mikayla to benefit from that. Mikayla got the first of three injections that day.

Mikayla still had questions, so the nurse practitioner recommended this book. Mikayla bought it right away and read the whole thing that night. It took a couple of more weekly visits and TCA treatments, but the warts finally cleared up completely. Mikayla was incredibly relieved.

Because she had read this book and knew it was a possibility, Mikayla wasn't really surprised when, at the end of the semester, several new warts cropped us. Finals were stressful. She was living on Diet Coke and pizza during short breaks from her studies. She wasn't sleeping, and there certainly wasn't time for exercise. She visited the student health center again.

Coincidently, it was time for Mikayla's second Gardasil shot. She was glad to see the same nurse practitioner and explained that once finals were over, she was heading off to do a summer internship. Because weekly visits for TCA treatments were not an option, the nurse practitioner prescribed Aldara cream (Imiquimod) for Mikayla to use on her own.

Mikayla started right away, following the instructions carefully because she had read that, while the medicine was very effective, using too much could cause her skin to get very inflamed and even ulcerated. After about 6 weeks, her warts were gone.

Mikayla's second episode of warts was another learning experience (college is full of learning experiences, some of them really tough ones). She realized the outbreak had probably occurred because she had been taking such poor care of herself at the end of the semester. She vowed to get more organized and manage her time and studies better.

Mikayla stuck to a better sleep schedule and stopped pulling "all-nighters". She swore off all junk food and fast food and decided that fruits and vegetables were her new best friends. She joined a running club while she was away doing her internship and was surprised to find she loved it! This was definitely a form of exercise she could keep up with back at school, no matter how crazy her schedule got.

Mikayla also started keeping a journal. It was really therapeutic for her to write about the ups and downs of college life. She tried very hard to end each entry by listing three things she was grateful for. This practice really helped her cultivate a more positive outlook on life.

Mikayla never had another episode of genital warts. Things didn't work out with Trey, and when she started dating someone new the next semester, she took things really slowly. Before she took things to the next level, she knew she was going to have to have "the talk" with her boyfriend and tell him about the warts. She really liked this guy, and after a few months of dating, she finally told him about her condition. He was really understanding about it and told Mikayla he wasn't too worried because his mom had made him take Gardasil before he left for college!

Chapter 4: Coping with HPV

If you have a positive HPV diagnosis, this is surely a difficult time for you. Whether you have been diagnosed with genital warts or had an abnormal Pap test, you probably have many questions and fears, such as:

"How did I get HPV?"

"Is this infection going to go away?"

"Will I get cervical cancer?"

"How is this going to affect my relationships and my sex life?"

It is common to have an emotional response to your diagnosis. Follow the following advice to keep your emotions in check and deal with your HPV diagnosis in the healthiest way possible.

Don't obsess about things you can't change

Decide to spend your energy only on things that will help you move forward. It is not productive to spend time wondering about when you got infected with HPV, or by whom. The bottom line is that you will never know for sure. Remember that HPV infection is very common. Most people with this condition, particularly men, have no idea they are infected. Whether you did or did not use condoms does not matter, because they do not provide 100% protection from this type of infection.

You may also be tremendously angry or embarrassed because you believe your HPV was a result of infidelity. However, a recent diagnosis of HPV does not necessarily mean that you or your partner has been unfaithful. This is even applicable to long-term relationships that span many years because it is possible to have HVP for a very, very long time without ever knowing it.

If you have good reason to suspect infidelity, know that this sort of relationship problem can be intensely stressful. You may need to get help from a counselor or pastor to help you work through your pain. Don't hesitate to get help. As you will learn in Chapter 10, managing stress is important for fighting HPV.

"But what my HPV infection was due to my own poor choices?"

People make mistakes. Forgive yourself as quickly as you can and spend your energy making better choices going forward!

Follow your health care provider's recommendations

In order to have the best possible outcomes from your HPV infection, it is important to follow your health care provider's advice.

- Follow your treatment instructions exactly. Use medications according to the prescribed schedule—don't miss days or doses.

- If your doctor recommends treatment, make sure you understand all of the options, risks, and benefits of the procedure. Also, be sure that you know how to take care of yourself afterward, and exactly what your schedule for follow-up care will be.

- Keep your follow-up appointments. If your health care provider wants you to return in a week to see if your treatment has been successful, be there. If you need to have another Pap test in 6 or 12 months, mark your calendar and get it done on time. Many studies have shown that diagnoses of cervical cancer are often associated with patient non-compliance. Don't let this happen to you!

- If you undergo a procedure for treatment, make sure you follow all of the post-procedure instructions. Refrain from intercourse for the recommended period of time. Attend your follow-up visit(s). Make

sure you understand any pathology reports
and when you need to return for another Pap
or HPV test.

Focus on what you can do

There are many actions you can take to help your
body fight an HPV infection, which will be discussed
in Part Two of this book. Your health care provider
may have already counseled you about these actions -
though some of them may be new to you. Read Part
Two of this book and discover how you can
incorporate this advice into your life. It's time to...

FIGHT BACK!

PART TWO:

Fight Back!

Chapter 5: Fighting an HPV Infection

Part Two of this book focuses on what you can do to maximize your chances for the best possible outcome of your HPV infection. That means:

- Minimizing recurrence of genital warts

- Having CIN 1 changes regress from your cervix

- Clearing high-risk strain infections of HPV

- Treating CIN 2 or 3 with no recurrence of symptoms

The natural history of your HPV infection depends on how well your immune system works to mount a response to the viral invasion. Specifically, it is up to your body to coordinate a cell-mediated immune (CMI) response:

- Your body activates cells called macrophages to recognize the HPV infection and calls special white blood cells called T-lymphocytes into action.

- Cytotoxic T-lymphocytes, once activated, recognize and directly kill cells that are infected with HPV with proteins known as cytokines and interferons.

- Cytokines also call other immune cells into action to fight the infection.

Failure to develop effective CMI to clear or control your HPV infection can result in a persistent infection. If high-risk strains of HPV are present, you face an increased risk of progressing to CIN 3 and invasive cervical cancer.

Many of the strategies in Part Two of this book are focused on making sure your immune system can function in the best way possible to fight back against HPV! Be sure to read every chapter and consider how you can incorporate this advice into your life.

Chapter 6: Stop Smoking Now!

If you are a smoker and are infected with high-risk HPV, you are twice as likely to develop CIN on your cervix. Tobacco smoke is a very well-established co-factor to HPV in the development of invasive cervical cancers. Also, if you are infected with HPV 6 or 11, you are at increased risk of developing genital warts and experiencing recurrences of warts. If you are a smoker, the most important thing that you MUST do to fight HPV is to STOP SMOKING NOW!

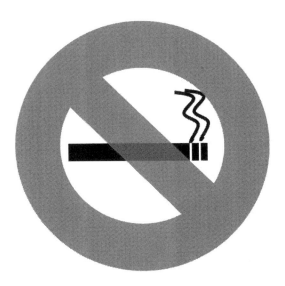

Why does smoking make infection with HPV so much worse? Well, one reason is that nicotine inhibits the immune response to HPV. Remember that the immune system kills cells that are infected with HPV and limits your formation of precancerous cells. Anything that impairs the immune system has a negative impact on your body's ability to fight HPV. Depending upon your type of HPV infection (low-risk or high-risk), this can lead to outbreaks of genital warts, a persistent HPV infection, and progression to precancerous abnormalities.

Second, carcinogenic tobacco by-products are found in the cervical mucus of women who smoke. These carcinogens amplify the effect of HPV infection within cervical cells. Researchers believe that these toxins damage the DNA of cervical cells and act as an accomplice to HPV in the development of cancerous changes.

A study done at the University of Washington showed that, within two years of having quit smoking, women's risk of cervical cancer declined to the level of women who had never smoked! This is good evidence that, even if you are a smoker with an HPV infection, your ultimate outcome will be much better if you stop smoking today. Isn't that a great motivation for kicking the habit?

Quitting smoking is not easy. Nicotine, the drug found in tobacco, is highly addictive and creates a powerful physical, mental, and emotional dependence. Most people have very unpleasant withdrawal symptoms when they quit. However, these can be managed with good planning. You can do it!

Entire books have been written on the topic of quitting smoking. It is not possible to do the topic justice here, but I will offer some basic advice for you to consider. I will also include a list of online resources you can check out.

Five Quit Smoking Tips:

- Pick a quit date. Now that you know how important quitting smoking is to fighting HPV, decide on a date—sooner rather than later.— on which you will completely stop smoking. Putting it off lessens the chances you will be successful. Make sure to choose a day that will not be very busy or stressful. Avoid quitting on a day when you will be particularly tempted to smoke (for instance, a day of the week you hang out with friends who are smokers). Circle this date on the calendar.

- Set up your support system. Let these people know you are planning to quit and that you want to be accountable to them in your effort. Choose people who will be supportive— people who really want to see you make this positive change. Let them know how they can help:

  - Keep you away from cigarettes

- Distract you with non-smoking activities

- Put up with you when you are grouchy

- Offer consistent support and encouragement

- Start cutting back as you approach your quit date. This is especially important if you are a heavy smoker. If you quit abruptly, you are likely to be very miserable.

- Have a plan to cope. Withdrawal from addiction can be very difficult, and you need to plan what you are going to do instead of smoking. Some ideas include:

  - chewing gum

  - biting on a toothpick

  - drinking water to flush the toxins

  - chewing whole cloves

  There are many different nicotine replacement products, and a number of drugs that have been proven effective in increasing your chances of success. Some are available over the counter, and some require a trip to your health care provider. Short term use of these products may be your key to success.

- Get active! Move! Exercise is a great way to help you avoid situations that make you want to smoke. Smoking cessation has been associated with weight gain, so moving your body will also help you stay thin. Besides that, it is a great way to celebrate your heart and lungs being clear of cigarette smoke!

Quit Smoking Resources:

Websites

- SMOKEFREE.gov – This site offers advice to help you quit, quizzes to assess readiness, a quit plan, and a place to sign up to receive encouraging texts. You will also discover insights into managing your weight through healthy eating and exercise.

- CANCER.org – The American Cancer Society offers a variety of related topics for consideration, including assistance in setting a quit date and steps for long-term success.

- HELPGUIDE.org – This site offers a "START" plan and discusses several symptoms and coping methods.

- WHYQUIT.com – This site offers 200+ videos, 2 free e-books, and a supportive community.

- LUNG.org - The American Lung Association has an area called the Quitter's Circle that offers important information on smoking cessation. It also offers insight into workplace wellness and tobacco-free campuses, as well as a variety of other tools.

- CDC.gov – This government site offers information about preparing to quit and getting support along the way.

iPhone and Android Apps

- LIVESTRONG MyQuit Coach helps you develop and track a personalized plan for either quitting smoking cold turkey or using a step-down approach.

- Quit It Lite is a motivational program that helps you track your goals by focusing on what you have not done—that is, the cigarettes you didn't smoke!

- QuitNow! helps you to manage the anxiety you experience when quitting. It helps break down the process of quitting into baby steps. It also gives you positive feedback as you progress about how you are helping your health (and your wallet).

- Quit Smoking helps you gradually cut back on your smoking. It provides statistical data that adjusts to your smoking pattern. You can watch your progress with each passing day!

Julia's Fight –HPV 16

Julia was at work when her gynecologist called with her Pap results. Because Julia is over 30, her doctor said she was going to do co-testing this year (combining a Pap smear with an HPV test).

Julia's doctor said that her Pap results had come back normal, but that her HPV test was positive for type 16 HPV, a type that is associated with cervical cancer. She told Julia to come back to her doctor's office and have a colposcopy.

Julia was worried. She thought, "Colposcopy? My sister had one of those. Isn't that what they do when they think someone has cervical cancer? Why would I need that if my Pap results are normal?"

Her doctor told her, "While Pap tests are good tests, they aren't perfect. 1 out of 10 women who are positive for HPV 16 or 18 may have a cervical disease that was missed by a Pap test. I'd like to do a colposcopy just to make sure. If we find any precancerous changes, we can treat them right away." She scheduled an appointment for Julia to come into her office.

That night at home, Julia lay in her bed thinking and worrying about what her doctor had told her. It had been a difficult year. She had gotten a divorce, moved into a new house, gone back to work at a job she did not love—and now this!

Julia had HPV that might cause cancer! Yikes! She wondered if her ex's infidelity had anything to do with it. She was angry, scared, worried, and tired of it all. Why did everything have to be so hard? When would things get better? She got out of bed and went to the back porch to smoke—a habit from back in her college days that she had restarted recently in an effort to deal with all the stresses in her life.

A week later, she had her colposcopy. Her gynecologist said that she did not see anything that looked worrisome. She told Julia that recent studies had shown that it was a good idea to take a couple of biopsies from her cervix even though everything looked good, so she had taken a few samples for good measure.

Later that week, Julia got her results—one of the biopsies showed a low-grade cervical epithelial neoplasia called CIN 1. Julia's doctor explained that this was additional confirmation of her HPV infection, and a sign that it was causing some mild abnormalities in the cells on her cervix.

However, Julia's doctor did not recommend any treatment at this time, to give Julia's body some time to see if it could heal on its own. She talked about certain actions Julia could take to get better naturally, such as stopping smoking and developing a strong immune system. She said that at Julia's next annual exam, she should repeat both her Pap and HPV tests. She also stressed the importance of having that exam exactly 12 months from now.

At first, Julia was terrified. "I'm going to get cervical cancer!" she thought over and over again. Panicked, she called her sister, who had been through something similar a few years ago.

Julia's sister calmed her down, as always. A couple days later, she sent Julia this book and advised that she read every word. Julia did read it that very night and decided it was time to make some changes.

First and foremost, Julia knew she had to stop smoking for good. She set a quit date and mapped out a plan to cut back her nicotine intake over a couple of weeks.

Julia knew that she must make other lifestyle changes to help to help her immune system fight back against HPV. Her stress level had been off the charts for at least a year, and that had to end. It was time to let go of some things. She had to move past her divorce and find a job she enjoyed.

Julia joined a divorce support group and met some really nice women who were going through many of the same things she was experiencing. It was so calming to have a chance to talk about her struggles and know that she was not alone. She really bonded with a couple of the women, and they started getting together outside of the group once a week to go walking at a local park. Julia found that she enjoyed being outside and started walking on her own nearly every night. One of the women also gave her a lead on a job opening that sounded interesting.

Little by little, Julia made important changes in her life, inspired by the book her sister had given her. She began taking a multivitamin with 600 mcg of 5 methyl-tetrahydrofolate (5-MTHF) and made it her goal to have five servings of vegetables every day. She also started going to a yoga class that incorporated meditation for some additional stress-relief. As Julia's stress level started coming down, her sleep improved. She no longer stayed up late, worrying and smoking.

By the time her next annual exam rolled around, Julia felt confident she was doing everything she possibly could to fight back against her HPV infection. Her doctor commented on how much happier Julia looked and commended her on kicking the smoking habit.

Julia was overjoyed when she got the letter in the mail telling her that both her Pap and HPV tests had come back negative! She resolved to maintain all the good health habits she had worked so hard to create during the past year.

Chapter 7: Limit Sexual Partners

As discussed in Part 1 of this book, having multiple sexual partners is a risk factor for HPV. Limiting your number of sexual partners is not only important when you are trying to prevent HPV, but it is also important after you have been diagnosed. Consider the following:

- There are many types of HPV, and a new partner may carry a strain that is different than the strain causing your current infection.

- It is usually not possible to know if a new partner has an HPV infection unless he/she discloses a history of previous infection or genital warts.

- Condoms are not completely effective at protecting you from HPV. HPV can infect areas not covered by the condom. It is correct, however, that consistent condom use can lower your chances of getting HPV and other STDs. There are also other benefits to condom use, as discussed in Chapter 8.

- Exposure to other strains of HPV may further tax your immune system and make it harder for your body to fight your infection.

It is best to have sex with just one person who only has sex with you! If you are actively being treated for genital warts, it is best to refrain from sex entirely until the warts are gone.

Handling a new relationship

Remember, having HPV means that you, like so many other people, have been exposed to a very common virus. Infection with HPV is not a reflection on you, your character, or your values! When you tell a new partner about your HPV infection, you should not consider it a "confession" or an "apology". It's simply a fact—something you're living with and coping with. You are not different from many other people.

With a new relationship, it's a good idea to date for a while and allow non-sexual aspects of your relationship to develop. You need to get to know one another and become close. You will know when the time is right to discuss your HPV infection. Make sure you are honest and share the facts about HPV, so your partner can understand your condition.

Remember that, for most people, HPV is harmless and does not result in visible symptoms or health consequences.

Chapter 8: Use Condoms

News flash! Using condoms can promote clearance of HPV and regression of the CIN lesions.

"How can this be? Didn't you just say that condoms offer limited protection against HPV infection? If that is the case, then how can condoms be helpful in getting rid of HPV?"

Keep reading to find out!

The Evidence

Two Norwegian studies recruited women with HPV infections that manifested as CIN 2 and CIN 3. Rather than receiving any treatment for their CIN, they were observed very closely over time, and their behaviors and outcomes were assessed.

In these studies, women whose partners used condoms had a much greater chance of clearing their HPV infections and having their CIN regress without any treatment. In fact, the odds of clearance and regression were 3-4 times greater for condom users than non-users. (This study also showed that smokers were much less likely to have a spontaneous clearance of HPV or a regression of CIN—more proof that smoking cessation is critical!)

The Theories

The most common theory for why condom use may be helpful AFTER someone has been infected with HPV is that condoms reduce the repeated exposure of the cervical surface to HPV. By interrupting exposure, the immune system is able to focus on the existing infection and mount its strongest defense possible.

A second theory centers on the belief that natural substances called prostaglandins, which are found in semen, have a strong immunosuppressive effect. Condom use keeps the surface of the cervix from being exposed to these prostaglandins, which may in turn impede the immune system from fighting HPV.

A third (very speculative) theory is that the latex in condoms stimulates a cellular immune response that promotes HPV clearance.

Whatever the mechanism, it is clear that condoms can be beneficial in fighting HPV. Women with HPV, particularly those who have been diagnosed with CIN, should present this information to their partners and encourage them to use condoms. They should discuss a study in the Netherlands that showed that men whose partners had CIN were often found to have HPV lesions on their penis when inspected under high magnification, and that those lesions were more likely to go away if they used condoms. It may take some convincing, but if your partner cares about you and your health, they will probably agree to use condoms in order to give you a chance to heal. You are worth it!

Chapter 9: Folate/Folic Acid

Folate is the term used to describe a group of B-vitamins also known as B9. Folic acid refers to a synthetic form of B9 that is commonly used in supplements and to fortify food.

Folic acid helps the body make healthy new cells. It is very important for women planning a pregnancy because it has been shown to prevent major birth defects like spina bifida (failure for the spinal column to close) and anencephaly (failure of the brain to develop).

A number of studies have explored the role that folic acid plays in the natural history of HPV infections. Researchers at the University of Alabama at Birmingham demonstrated that women with higher blood levels of folate have a much lower likelihood of becoming infected with high-risk HPV and have a lower risk of developing persistent high-risk HPV infections. Also, they showed that women with adequate levels of folate are more likely to clear away high-risk HPV infections. Women with low levels of folate were twice as likely to have high-grade CIN. Also, women with low folate and infection with HPV 16 were nine times more likely to have CIN 2 and CIN 3!

How does folate work on a molecular level? DNA contains combinations of four molecules (called "nucleotides"): cytosine, guanine, thymine, and adenine. DNA methylation refers to the addition of a methyl (CH_3) group to the cytosine or guanine nucleotides. DNA methylation plays an important part in the development of cancer. In cervical cells infected with HPV and with low folic acid levels, DNA methylation occurs aberrantly and cancer-causing genes become methylated and promote cancerous changes. When folate is present in adequate amounts, aberrant methylation does not occur.

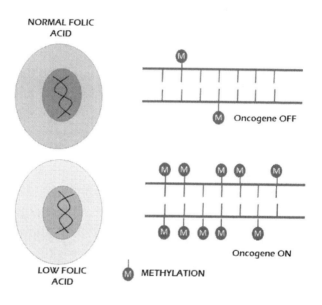

Excellent natural sources of dietary folate include vegetables such as:

- romaine lettuce

- spinach

- asparagus

- mustard greens

- broccoli

- cauliflower

- beans

- nuts

Because folic acid is so important to preventing birth defects, many foods are enriched with folic acid, such as:

- breakfast cereals

- breads

- flours

- pasta

- white rice

Interestingly, it is harder for the body to use natural folate, so we can't be sure that eating foods that contain natural folate will provide the amounts we need. This is one of those rare cases where supplements are probably the best way to go. If you follow a low-carb or gluten-free diet, this is particularly important; these diets do not include many of the foods that are fortified with folate.

It is a good idea to take a multivitamin or supplement to ensure you are getting enough folic acid. You should aim for 400-800 micrograms (mcg) a day. Be careful, though, and know that more is not better; in fact, too much folic acid has been associated with certain risks. It seems that some people have a hard time metabolizing folic acid into its useful form, and the presence of high levels of unmetabolized folic acid in the blood has been associated with cancer. Some experts are now suggesting that, if folate supplementation is needed, it should be in the form of 5-methyl-tetrahydrofolate (5-MTHF) because it is used more easily by the body.

Chapter 10: Reduce Stress

Fighting an HPV infection involves optimizing your immune system so your body can mount an adequate cell-mediated immune response.

There is abundant evidence that chronic stress takes a significant toll on your immune system. In fact, scientists have coined the term "psychoneuroimmunology" to describe how one's state of mind impacts the immune system's ability to fight infection.

Acute stress results in a flight-or-fight response, a mechanism designed to help you survive an attack. Your adrenal glands flood your bloodstream with adrenaline and cortisol to call your body's resources to action. The result is a burst of increased energy and alertness that helps you cope with a threat to your survival. In the short term, blood is directed away from your gut and into your muscles and limbs. Your awareness intensifies, your perception of pain diminishes, and your immune system mobilizes and activates.

But what happens when stress is prolonged? In that case, cortisol remains in the bloodstream for a long period of time and wears down the immune system. It actually suppresses the function of your T-cells (which are pivotal to cell-medicated immunity). Cortisol keeps your T-cells from proliferating and impairs their ability to recognize the chemical signals that tell them how to do their job.

As a result, the body is less able to fight infections, including HPV infections. If you want your immune system to do the best possible job of fighting your HPV infection, then you simply <u>must</u> manage your stress.

Stress Management 101

Everyone has stress at some point in their life. Sometimes it is brief and situational, like when taking a test. At other times, it is persistent and complex, in situation such as:

- Relationship problems, especially divorce
- Changing jobs and/or moving
- Coping with a family member's ailing health
- A difficult work environment
- Fighting illness (including an HPV infection!)

In a perfect world, you would identify the things that cause your stress and just get rid of them. Unfortunately, it is often not possible to eliminate all of your stressors. I mean, really—who can just quit their job just because it is stressful, or ditch their family because they make you crazy? In many circumstances, managing stress means learning and practicing skills that can help you cope with difficult situations.

Exercise

Exercise is one of the very best ways to cope with stress. The physical benefits of exercise have long been established, and physicians almost always encourage their patients to stay physically active.

Exercise is considered vital for maintaining mental fitness, and it also reduces stress. Studies show that it is very effective at reducing fatigue, improving alertness and concentration, and enhancing your overall cognitive function. Exercise reduces your body's stress hormone levels, such as adrenaline and cortisol. It also stimulates the production of endorphins, brain chemicals that are the body's natural painkillers and mood elevators. Endorphins are responsible for the "runner's high" and for the feelings of relaxation and optimism that accompany a good workout.

In moderation, exercise is good for the immune system. It promotes good circulation, which allows the cells and substances of your immune system to move through the body freely and do their job efficiently.

Too much exercise, however, can be bad for the immune system. Very intense workouts are physical stressors that can increase cortisol and suppress the immune system, leaving you less able to fight infection. In other words, 30 to 60 minutes of moderate exercise (such as walking or jogging 4-5 days a week) is a great way to manage stress and boost your immune system. However, relentless, excessively intense workouts can be counterproductive.

Meditate

Research has shown that regular meditation and relaxation can significantly reduce your stress to manageable and healthy levels. Through meditation, you can learn to focus and quiet your mind, and let go of the negative thoughts and feelings associated with stress. People who practice mediation also show measurable physical improvements: slower heart rates, reduced metabolisms, and lower levels of adrenaline and cortisol!

Meditation has also been shown to boost the immune system. A recent study demonstrated that, after two months of weekly meditation training, 48 biotech workers had significantly higher levels of antibodies than they did at the beginning of the study. They also had higher antibodies than the "control group" (coworkers who didn't meditate).

You may think that meditation involves sitting on the floor and chanting "Om". While some forms of meditation involve these techniques, there are many ways to meditate.

One popular method is known as Mindfulness-Based Stress Reduction (MBSR). This technique uses both breath awareness and a body scan. Breath awareness is as simple as it sounds—you focus your attention on breathing in and out. A body scan is a process of focusing your attention on your physical body, starting at your toes and working your way up through your body.

MBSR techniques can help you develop a heightened sense of awareness and release your mental and physical stresses. This type of meditation may be performed while seated, laying down, or even while walking.

There are lots of other types of meditation you can explore. Even prayer and yoga can be forms of meditation.

Be Grateful

Research has shown that people who feel grateful are happier, more satisfied with their lives, less stressed, and healthier than those who do not. Gratitude means being appreciative of the positive things in your life rather than feeling bad about the negative things.

Gratitude breeds optimism, which has been linked to better immune function. In a study of first-year law students under stress at the University of Utah, it was found that students who were characterized as optimistic maintained higher numbers of immune cells in their blood.

Here are some ways to cultivate gratitude:

Keep a gratitude journal

Start a daily ritual of writing down things for which you are grateful.

- Decide to write down at least 3-5 things daily (even on your worst days).

- Be specific. Instead of "I am grateful for my health", write "I am grateful for my healthy body that allowed me to take a walk in the park today."

- Writing down the positive aspects of negative events, like "I was disappointed that things didn't work out in this relationship, but now I have time to focus on myself and my own needs."

Gratitude journaling right before bed has been associated with improved sleep. Researchers found that people who jotted down what they were grateful for 15 minutes before sleeping fell asleep faster and stayed asleep longer. You'll find out more in Chapter 11 about how important sleep is to fighting your HPV infection.

Count your blessings

Spend some time each day reflecting on what went right each day. Try to do this at a specific time each day. Also, try doing this when something does not go right, or when you feel like complaining. This practice fosters a healthy, positive mindset.

Pray

If you are religious, prayer is a terrific way to express gratitude. In a study at Bowling Green University, researchers instructed one group of migraine sufferers to meditate 20 minutes a day, repeating a religious affirmation: "God is good. God is peace. God is love." The other group used a nonspiritual mantra: "Grass is green. Sand is soft." The researchers found that the group using the religious affirmations had decreased headaches and increased pain tolerance. The really amazing part of this study was that the results were NOT dependent upon the religious beliefs of the participants!

Reach out

It can be difficult to manage stress when you feel isolated or alone. Reaching out to others can be very therapeutic.

- Lean on your family and friends, and talk about your stressors. Do not just focus on the negatives; Have your supporters help you problem-solve and be optimistic.

- Take part in community, religious, or other social events. Feeling like a part of a group helps breed positive feelings.

- Volunteer your time. Focusing on the needs and challenges of others can help you develop a different perspective on your situation.

Chapter 11: Get Some Sleep

It is well established that people who don't get enough sleep are susceptible to chronic disease. Our bodies have natural sleep-wake cycles known as circadian rhythms. Our internal clock is synced with many of our bodily functions, including—of course—our immune system.

When we get enough sleep, our immune system functions well; when we are sleep-deprived, our immune system becomes overactive. If you are trying to eradicate a persistent HPV infection, this may sound like a good thing, but it is not. This type of immune response is an inflammatory one, not a healing one.

Research has shown that sleep deprivation, especially long-term sleep deprivation, activates inflammation—an action of the immune system which is responsible for things like allergies, asthma, and other chronic illnesses (like heart disease and diabetes). The protective functions of the immune system (such as fighting viral infections) are suppressed when the immune system is in inflammatory mode, allowing many infections to progress unchecked.

During sleep of adequate duration, our immune system enters healing mode. The inflammatory response declines and cell-mediated immunity kicks in and is able to perform critical functions like eradicating HPV and healing CIN.

Are you getting enough sleep?

Take the Maas Robbins Alertness Questionnaire to assess whether you are getting enough sleep. Simply answer yes/no the following questions:

- I often need an alarm clock in order to wake up at the appropriate time.

- It's often a struggle for me to get out of bed in the morning.

- Weekday mornings, I often hit the snooze bar several times.

- I often feel tired and stressed out during the week.

- I often feel moody and irritable, and little things upset me.

- I often have trouble concentrating and remembering.

- I often feel slow with critical thinking, problem-solving, and being creative.

- I need caffeine to get going in the morning or make it through the afternoon.

- I often wake up craving junk food, sugars, and carbohydrates.

- I often fall asleep watching TV.

- I often fall asleep in boring meetings or lectures, or in warm rooms.

- I often fall asleep after heavy meals, or after a low dose of alcohol.

- I often fall asleep while relaxing after dinner.

- I often fall asleep within five minutes of getting into bed.

- I often feel drowsy while driving.

- I often sleep extra hours on the weekends.

- I often need a nap to get through the day.

- I have dark circles around my eyes.

- I fall asleep easily when watching movies.

- I rely on energy drinks or over-the-counter medications to keep me awake.

Did you answer "yes" to four or more of these statements? If so, you probably need more sleep!

How much sleep should you be getting?

In the table below, you will find recommendations from the experts at the National Sleep Foundation on how much sleep you should be getting.

National Sleep Foundation Recommendations

Age	Recommended	May be appropriate	Not recommended
Teenagers 14-17	8-10 hours	7 hours 11 hours	Less than 7 hours More than 11 hours
Young Adults 18-25 years	7-9 hours	6 hours 10 -11 hours	Less than 6 hours More than 11 hours
Adults 26-64 years	7-9 hours	6 hours 10 hours	Less than 6 hours More than 10 hours
Older Adults ≥ 65 years	7-8 hours	5 - 6 hours 9 hours	Less than 5 hours More than 9 hours

Here are a few tips on how to get more sleep:

- Set a consistent bedtime and stick with it. Optimally, this is the time you should go to bed every night of the week.

- Banish screens before bed. The light that emanates from television, phone, and computer screens can interfere with your ability to sleep. Power down your devices an hour before you go to bed to signal your body that it's time for sleep.

- Get exercise during the day. Moderate exercise that raises your heart rate can help you sleep better. However, don't exercise right before bed; this will have the opposite effect.

- Curb caffeine in the afternoon. Make it a rule to steer clear of Starbucks after lunch!

- Create a wind-down ritual before bed. A warm bath is very conducive to sleep. Meditation or journaling before sleep is also a great practice. Reading is also okay if the book isn't a page-turner that keeps you awake!

Chapter 12: Other Nutritional Weapons

There are lots of epidemiology studies demonstrating that the consumption of fruits and vegetables rich in antioxidants and other nutrients can lower your risk of cancer. Let's discuss a few key nutrients, and how can optimize your arsenal in the fight against HPV!

Fruit and Vegetable Intake

Several studies have examined the impact of the intake of fruits and vegetables on the natural history of HPV. A low intake of fruits and vegetables has been associated with HPV persistence. Similarly, studies have shown that low intake of cruciferous vegetables like cabbage, broccoli, and cauliflower has been associated with progression to high-grade CIN.

Let this inspire you to nourish your body with natural, healthy foods!

Beta-carotenes and Retinoid

Beta-carotene is the natural precursor of vitamin A and is found in green leafy vegetables. Studies have shown a protective effect of beta-carotenes on HPV persistence, but the strength of the association is not great. Likewise, a number of studies have looked at the influence of beta-carotenes on the regression of CIN lesions, but the results have not been impressive.

Studies of supplementation with retinoid (vitamin A) have not shown it to impact clearance of HPV but have demonstrated a reduced risk of CIN development. The amount of vitamin A in your diet (and a balanced multivitamin) is probably sufficient. High doses of retinoid have been associated with birth defects, so be careful not to over-do it.

I3C and DIM

Indole-3-carbinol (I3C) and its congener diindolylmethane (DIM) are derived from cruciferous vegetables such as broccoli and cabbage. Studies indicate that I3C has the potential to prevent and even treat a number of common cancers, especially those that are estrogen-related. In a double-blind, placebo-controlled study, 30 patients with biopsy-confirmed CIN II and III were randomized to receive a placebo or 200 or 400 mg oral I3C daily for 12 weeks. Three patients did not complete the study. The results:

- None of the 10 patients in the placebo group had complete regression of the CIN

- Four of eight patients in the 200-mg/day group had complete regression of the CIN.

- Four of nine in the 400-mg/day group had complete regression of the CIN.

I3C is easily available over the counter as a supplement, or simply by eating 4-5 servings of cruciferous family vegetables a day.

Turmeric

Turmeric is a spice commonly used in Indian cooking. Curcumin is the substance that gives the spice tumeric its bright yellow color. It has been found to have powerful anti-inflammatory and anti-oxidant properties as well as antiviral properties. Researchers in New Delhi found that curcumin inhibits the expression of oncoproteins in HPV infected cells. It also promotes programmed cell death in those cells and enhances tumor suppressing proteins. Curcumin is currently being investigated as a treatment for HPV-related oral cancers and cervical cancer. While there is no evidence yet to suggest the curcumin is clinically effective, some naturopathic experts have suggested there may benefits to taking 400-800 mg of curcumin supplements on a daily basis if you have an HPV infection. Note - turmeric has been associated with decreased fertility, so if you are trying to become pregnant you should speak to your health care provider.

All-Star Vegetables

Try to eat these every day!

Broccoli

Broccoli is the king of the cruciferous vegetable family. Its close relatives include brussel sprouts, cauliflower, and cabbage. As mentioned above, it is high in I3C and is also a good natural source of folate. A cup of broccoli has as much vitamin C as an orange!

However, be aware that some cooking methods can diminish the health benefits of broccoli. In fact, boiling can leach up to 90% of the valuable nutrients from this vegetable! Steaming, roasting, stir-frying, and microwaving tend to preserve the nutrients in broccoli.

Spinach

Popeye had it right! Spinach is good for you. As a dark leafy green, spinach is a great source of carotenoids and vitamin K and is a good source of folate. One cup of raw spinach contains 27 calories, 0.86 grams of protein, 30 milligrams of calcium, 0.81 grams of iron, 24 milligrams of magnesium, 167 milligrams of potassium, 2813 IUs of vitamin A, and 58 micrograms of folate.

You can eat spinach raw in a salad or cooked as a side dish. It can also be included in pasta dishes, soups, casseroles, and smoothies.

Kale

Kale is both a leafy green and a cruciferous vegetable! It is chock-full of the essential vitamins A, C, and K, as well as minerals like copper, potassium, iron, manganese, and phosphorus. Because it is cruciferous, it is a natural source of I3C. A cup of fresh kale has only about 40 calories, but packs in almost 3 grams of protein.

One cup of cooked kale has over 1000% more vitamin C than a cup of cooked spinach, and unlike spinach, kale's oxalate content is very low, which means that the calcium and iron in kale are highly absorbable in the human digestive system.

Kale can be enjoyed raw in salads, sandwiches, or wraps. It can also be braised, boiled, sautéed, or added to soups, casseroles, or smoothies. You can even make chips from it by tossing the leafy parts (minus the ribs) with oil and roasting them in the oven until crisp!

Bonnie's Fight – CIN 3

Bonnie had not had a physical exam in a while. Her husband had lost his job, and they had gone without health insurance for almost three years. Now that he had a new good job with benefits, Bonnie knew she needed to catch up on all of her health care needs—a Pap test, mammogram, cholesterol test, and a complete physical—the works!

About four years before, Bonnie had had a bad Pap test and a colposcopy which showed CIN 1. Her doctor had told her these were mild changes that would likely go away. They hoped that everything would be okay when she had her Pap test the next year. However, she'd never taken that Pap test because of her insurance situation. In the back of her mind, she had been worried about it.

Bonnie felt anxious when her doctor called her and said she needed to come in for another colposcopy that week. Her Pap had been read as "high-grade squamous intraepithelial lesion" (HSIL), which her doctor said was suggestive of possible high-grade precancerous cells. He said a colposcopy would help him determine what was really going on. Bonnie made an appointment for the following day. She did not sleep a wink that night.

The next day, Bonnie had her colposcopy. Her doctor placed a speculum into her vagina, just like he would when giving a Pap test. He used a magnifying scope called a colposcope to examine her cervix closely with a very bright light. He also used large cotton swabs to paint Bonnie's cervix with a vinegar solution. Bonnie thought that was really strange, but her doctor said it helped him to see her abnormal cells better.

Bonnie's doctor was really quiet during her colposcopy, and it seemed like he took forever just looking through the scope. He announced he was going to take a few biopsies. They were quick, and just felt like a big pinch. Afterward, he put a brown-orange paste called Monsel's on her cervix to stop the bleeding from the biopsies. He told her that the paste would come out and to expect it to be black and gunky. Although the procedure seemed endless to Bonnie, her doctor was done in less than 15 minutes. He told Bonnie he would call her in a few days when he got her pathology report.

Bonnie got the call, and the news wasn't great. Her doctor said the report showed she had high-grade precancerous cells, "cervical intraepithelial neoplasia 3", or "CIN 3". This meant there were areas on her cervix where precancerous changes spanned the entire thickness of the surface. The cells had not broken through the basement membrane, so it was not invasive cancer—yet.

If Bonnie's precancerous cells were not removed, over time, they could become invasive - a very serious condition. He recommended treatment with an in-office procedure called a LEEP. Bonnie was so upset that she really couldn't take it all in at that moment. The doctor said he understood, and that she should not worry because this treatment was very effective in preventing cervical cancer. He said that a nurse would call later to make an appointment, tell Bonnie what to expect, and answer any questions she had.

The nurse did call and explained everything that would be done in detail, and set up the appointment for the LEEP. Bonnie asked where she could read more about her condition, and the nurse recommended this book.

Bonnie's husband went to the doctor's office with her the day of the procedure. It was all really quite simple and actually took less time than the colposcopy. Again, her doctor used a speculum; this time it was made of plastic and had a port where he could attach a vacuum.

 Her doctor injected numbing medicine into her cervix and used a fine wire loop with an electric current running through it to cut away a thin layer of her cervix. The vacuum cleared away vapors released during the procedure. After that, he used electrocautery to control bleeding. He also put more of Monsel's paste on the cervix. The procedure was quick and relatively easy.

Bonnie was warned to call her doctor if she had any heavy bleeding in the next few weeks. She was told not to place anything in her vagina, such as tampons or douches, and not to have sex until a check-up visit in 4 weeks. She felt fine afterward and was relieved when the nurse called to tell her that the pathology report confirmed CIN 3, but that the margins were clear. This meant it was likely that all of her precancerous cells had been removed.

Bonnie was instructed that her four-week doctor's visit was just a quick check to confirm that her cervix had healed. Her next follow-up exam would be in 12 months. At that visit, they would do co-testing—both Pap and HPV tests. If either test was abnormal, a colposcopy would be repeated. If both were okay, then she'd have co-testing again in a year.

The abnormal cells were gone, but would the HPV go away? Bonnie discussed this issue with her doctor and told him she had read this book. They talked at length about the things she could work on before her next appointment.

Bonnie's stress level was much improved now that her husband's long unemployment had ended. Bonnie suspected that this might have contributed to the progression of her abnormal cells in those few years. The stress had been awful and became worse the longer it took her husband to find a new job.

Bonnie's doctor agreed that her chronic stress may have been a contributing factor to her illness. Bonnie promised to work hard on managing her day-to-day stress over the next year. She promised to exercise and work on her diet. She was planting a large garden that year, so there would be plenty of vegetables to eat.

Bonnie asked her doctor if she and her husband should use condoms, as suggested in Chapter 8 of this book. Bonnie had her tubes tied years ago, and she and her husband had been married a long time. She did not think he would be thrilled with the idea. Her doctor said that the studies on this issue had been small, but the results were compelling.

Although Bonnie's doctor could not say condom use was mandatory, he said it was something to consider. He said, "Let's say you and Mike use condoms for 4-6 months after this LEEP. If there is no sign of HPV at the next visit, will you regret it? If there is still HPV, will you at least feel you tried everything you could?" Bonnie agreed that this was an interesting way to think about the issue. She said she would talk to her husband about it.

Bonnie left the visit feeling hopeful. The LEEP had gone well, and she knew there were things she could do over the next year to increase her chances of clearing away her HPV infection once and for all. Despite the lapse in her health care, she was going to be okay!

Chapter 13: Prevention

If I already have HPV, isn't it too late to talk about prevention? The answer to this question is "NO!" It is not at all too late. Remember that there are different types of HPV: low-risk types that cause genital warts and low-grade CIN, as well as high-grade types that have the potential to cause cancer. Taking preventative measures, specifically practicing safe sex and getting vaccinated, can help you to avoid becoming infected with other types of HPV.

Preventing Transmission

If you know you have been infected with HPV, you must prevent transmission to your sexual partner(s)! Also, you want to reduce the risk of becoming infected with a new and different type of HPV.

Using barrier methods (condoms and dental dams) can reduce the risk of infection. Remember that protection cannot be 100% because HPV can be present in skin not covered by a condom or dental dam. You and your partner(s) will have agree on what risks you are comfortable with.

Vaccination

Vaccination is a safe and effective way to reduce the risk of both genital warts and cervical cancer. There are currently three HPV vaccines available in the United States:

- Cervarix – covers high-risk HPV types 16 and 18

- Gardasil – covers low-risk HPV types 6 and 11, as well as high-risk types 16 and 18

- Gardasil 9 – covers low-risk HPV types 6 and 11, as well as high-risk types 16, 18, 31, 33, 45, 52, and 58

The newest formulation, Gardasil 9, offers superior coverage. The studies leading to its approval indicated that in addition to protecting against the two types of low-risk HPV responsible for 90% of genital warts, it is able to protect against 85-90% of cervical cancers!

Who should get vaccinated against HPV?

HPV vaccination is recommended for 11 and 12-year-old girls. It is also recommended for girls and women age 13 through 26 years of age who have not yet been vaccinated or completed the vaccine series. It is also recommended that boys and men aged 11-26 get vaccinated.

Gardasil 9 is given as 3 injections over 6 months; the second dose comes 2 months after the first dose and the third dose comes 6 months after the first dose.

HPV vaccine will not treat an existing HPV infection. But as I said earlier, it can protect you from being infected by new HPV types. Talk to your health care provider about whether vaccination is right for you.

How safe are HPV Vaccines?

In short, very!

HPV vaccines, including the new one, have been tested in tens of thousands of people in the United States and many other countries before being approved for use. NO serious side effects have been shown to be caused by the vaccines. The most common problem, soreness at the site of the shot, is expected with vaccines because they stimulate the immune system.

More than 67 MILLION doses of HPV vaccine were given in the U.S. between 2006 and 2014. The FDA collects safety information on complaints of adverse effects after these vaccinations. The most frequent symptoms were fainting, dizziness, nausea, headache, fever, and hives. Also, patients experienced localized pain, redness, and swelling at the site of the injection. This is not very surprising.

Some more serious negative events were reported, but there was no pattern to the reports and no direct proof that the events were related to the vaccine—except for fainting. Sometimes needle-phobic people faint due to the stress of getting a shot, and may hit their head. It is now recommended that people sit down when getting an HPV vaccine.

The issue of HPV vaccination is monitored closely, and the evidence is overwhelming that the benefits of vaccination FAR outweigh any risks that may be involved.

Chapter 14: Putting It All Together

I have given you a lot of information about HPV and what you can do to have the best possible outcome in fighting your infection. Hopefully, you feel motivated that you can make a difference in your own care.

You really can get through this! Now is the time for you to put it all together and make a plan of action.

Step 1:

Understand what your health care provider wants you to do and DO IT!

- Know your diagnosis and treatment plan. Ask questions. What are the risks? Benefits? Alternatives? What should you expect?

- Know when you need to see your health care provider for a follow-up Pap test or exam. Make your appointment and mark it on your calendar. Arrange your school or work schedule, so you can keep your appointment.

- It's also a good idea to know what will come next. If your health care provider wants you to have a Pap test in 6 months, when will the next one be? Make sure you understand the entire plan. Ask questions! Even better, write down your questions before the appointment.

- If you have been given medication to use, follow the instructions exactly. Understand how often you are to use a medication and for how long. Know when or if you need to go back for a check-up after completing your treatment. What sort of side effects should you look out for? What should you do if they arise? Who should you call if you have questions after your appointment?

Step 2:

Figure out what actions from Part Two of this book you will take to fight HPV. Go through this book again and write down the good habits you plan to implement. Post this list somewhere you will see it daily, as a reminder of what you need to do! Consider this written list a commitment to yourself.

Step 3:

Make a step-by-step plan for each action you have committed to. Think about your motivations, the potential obstacles, and the actions and people that can help you be successful. What might your first steps be? For example:

- Stop Smoking

    - Decide how you are going to go about it

    - Set a quit date

    - Enlist support from family and friends

- Use Condoms

  - Buy condoms
  - Have a conversation with your partner about why condom use is important

- Increase Your Folate Levels

  - Stock your pantry and fridge with folate-rich foods
  - Buy a high-quality supplement

- Manage Your Stress

  - Identify the biggest causes of stress in your life
  - Schedule time for exercise
  - Get an app to help you meditate
  - Buy a journal and start writing

- Sleep Better

  - Establish a consistent bedtime to ensure you get enough sleep, and stick to it!
  - Create a night-time ritual to help you wind down and get to sleep fast

- Nutrition

  - Keep a food diary to track the quality of your diet (there's an app for that...)

- Buy more fruits and vegetables
- Consider an I3C supplement
- Visit a nutritionist for advice

Step 4:

Be positive! Your attitude really <u>can</u> make a difference.

If and when you have negative thoughts about HPV and your health, push them out of your head. Replace them with positive thoughts and remind yourself of the many things you can do to take care of yourself. Adopt the healthiest lifestyle you can, to strengthen your immune system.

Consider every good choice you make a victory. Stay strong and motivated!

And, as I have said over and over again...

FIGHT BACK!

Acknowledgements

First, I want to acknowledge all the women I have cared for in my clinical practice. Thank you for giving me your trust and allowing me to be a part of your health journey. Your questions and concerns were the inspiration for this book. I no longer provide direct patient care, but I remain committed to working every day toward better health for women - because of you.

Second, I want to acknowledge my daughter, Ruby. It has been a pure joy watching you develop into the amazing young woman that you are. Your drive and determination are astonishing. You truly are full of the light of God and your father and I are so blessed by you. I see you leading such a healthy and balanced life, and I know that the future holds many, many great things for you. I know it is supposed to be the other way around, but YOU inspire me.

Finally, and most importantly, I have to acknowledge my husband, Ken. You are my favorite editor, my love, my foundation - my everything. You support every crazy thing I want to do with gusto—even when I say things like, "I want to write a book."

I don't know how you do it. Don't stop.

About The Author

Laura McKain, MD is an obstetrician/gynecologist who received her medical degree from Georgetown University. 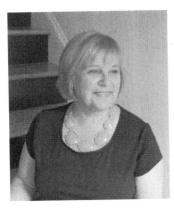 She had a busy and successful private practice for more than a dozen years before deciding to transition her career to clinical research. She is passionate about providing women with information about their health and draws from research from both conventional and alternative medicine. It is her opinion that lifestyle and nutrition are important factors in wellness and that healing should be approached holistically.

Dr. McKain lives in coastal North Carolina with her husband and daughter.

Made in the USA
Charleston, SC
21 May 2015